WHAT'S COOKING AT KATHY MORROW STUDIO

Two of my many loves in life are cooking and painting My cook book is seasoned with the stories that inspired my art.

My Diabetes and Gluten intolerance have led to creativity in the kitchen. The specialty foods available in stores today are abundant but expensive and not always tasty. Preservatives and artificial ingredients to enhance flavor such as "Natural Flavors" add unnecessary chemicals to our diets.

There is a list of my favorite ingredients and why I prefer using them.

I hope you enjoy this little book as much as I enjoyed writing it.

www.kathymorrowstudio.com

Written by Kathy Morrow

Copyright 2013
All Rights Reserved

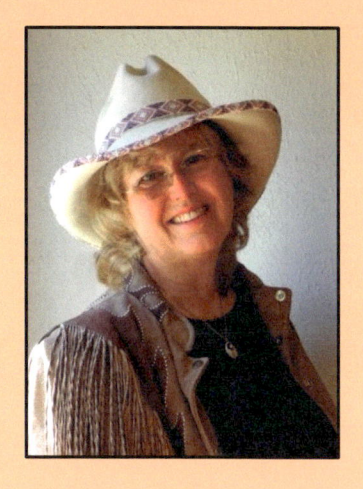

Kathy Morrow – Artist

   I like to paint a variety of subjects: Native American themes; Wildlife; Western themes with children and Santa; Desert flowers with Hummingbirds; Lions; Tigers; and Bears . . . Oh MY! I find there is beauty in everything and everyone. All of the people and animals in my art are real and my wild imagination sees stories everywhere. That used to get me in a lot of trouble in school when I was a kid and my Mom saved all the notes from my teachers saying "Kathy is a daydreamer". Thank Goodness that I finally found work where daydreaming paid off!

   Although, I have formal training in many mediums and paint with Acrylics on canvas in addition to Paintings on Clay Board, my greatest training has come from the School of Hard Knocks. I have spent a life time learning through discovery and experimenting with various techniques and materials. Each painting is my teacher.

   The School of Hard Knocks has taken me down other unexpected roads in life as well. Diabetes is rampant in our family and to complicate the diet regime some more, I developed intolerance to Gluten. This has led to more creativity to the kitchen. I wanted to share some of my favorite recipes with you and some of my favorite paintings too and of course the stories that inspired them.
Enjoy the Journey,
Kathy Morrow

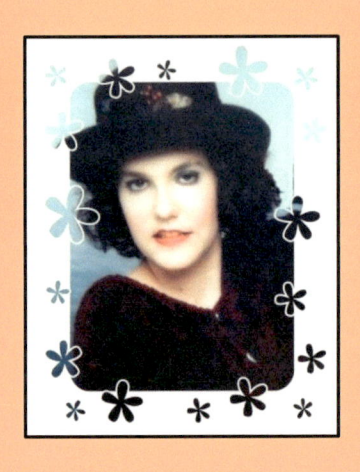

This book is dedicated to our daughter:
Stacy Lynn Morrow
1975 – 2000

(Cover Art)

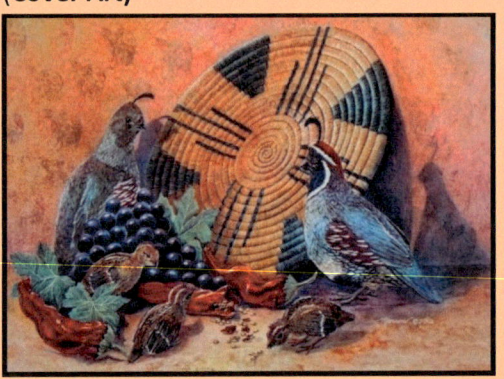

Mesilla Harvest   Limited Edition of 95
Signed and Numbered
Limited Edition Prints and Originals are available at www.KathyMorrowStudio.com

STORIES	RECIPES
1. Lobo Love	2. Pineapple Cranberry Upside-Down Cake
3. Still Waters	4. Almond Chocolate Chip Cake
5. On Gossamer Wings	6. Peanut Butter Chocolate Chip Cake
7. Do 'in 80	8. Banana Bread
9. Can You Hear Me Now?	10. Lemon Poppy Seed
11. Window of Opportunity The Mad Hatter	12. Spicy Carrot Cake
13. Pretty in Pink The Lady or The Tiger	14. Blueberry Coffee Cake
15. Sugar Bear	16. Pumpkin Nut Bread
17. Navajo Barbie	18. The Chocolate Lady's Cake
19. Santa's Secret	20. Chocolate Almond Cake
21. Tatanka Christmas	22. Zucchini Nut Bread
23. Horse Laugh	24. Apple Crumb Cake
25. Sky Hawk	26. Cranberry Nut Cake
27. Beep Beep	28. Orange Date Nut Bread
29. Cathy Williams Revealed	30. Waffles & Pancakes
31. Ghost Dancing	32. Cheesy Corn Bread
33. Apache Spirit Basket	34. Plain Sandwich Bread
35. Apache Spirit Pony	36. Parmesan Italian Bread
37. Mountain Spirit Pony	38. Sun Dried Tomato Bread
39. Horse Feathers	40. Mexican Salsa Bread
41. Give Me Wings	42. Plain Vanilla Cake
43. My Favorite Things	44. Author's Notes

1.

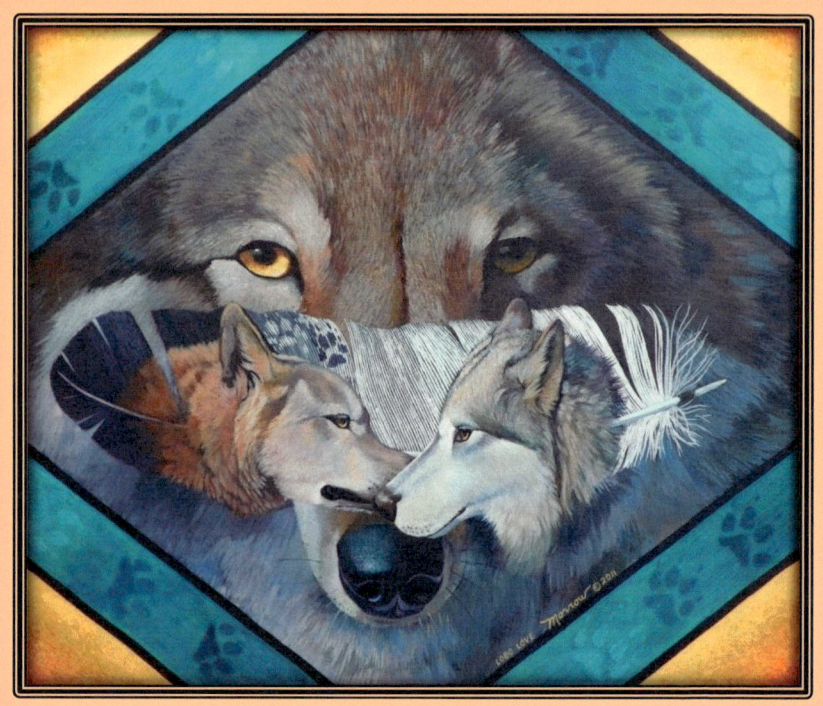

Lobo Love - The larger wolf is from the original Candy Kitchen Wolf Rescue Center, that is now called Wild Spirit Wolf Sanctuary. His name is Zeus and he was a little over a year old. He is guarding the two kissing wolves on the eagle feather.

   They are Manu and his mate Sequoia. Manu was severely abused by being tied in a yard to a tree and neglected. When he was brought to the rescue center, he was nearly dead. The Vet said he had not more than a week left. The people at the center worked with him for months, restoring his physical health and working on his mental health. Wolves, by nature are social animals and Manu wanted nothing to do with people or wolves. Over a long period of time, various female wolves were introduced to him and he chased them away until one day they brought a new female, Sequoia into his pen. She was an Alpha female and did not tolerate his attitude. There was a click and it was love at last for good old Manu. Now we know that behind every Manu is a good woman.

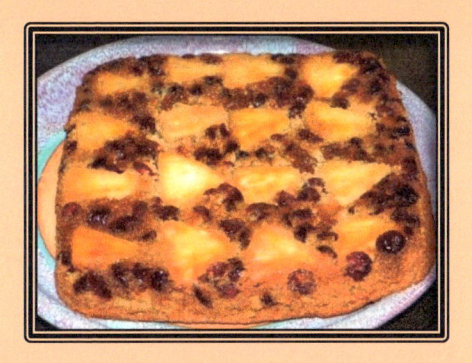

PINEAPPLE CRANBERRY UPSIDE DOWN CAKE

Pre-heat oven to 350 degrees

In a blender add the following and blend until smooth and creamy:

- 4 large Eggs
- 1 can - rinsed /drained Chick Peas (Garbanzo Beans) 15 oz. can
- 3/4 cup Coconut Palm Sugar
- 1 Tablespoon Vanilla Extract
- 2 teaspoons Cinnamon
- 2 teaspoons Baking Powder

Blend above ingredients thoroughly and pour OVER fruit arranged in the bottom of a 9 x 9 ceramic or Pyrex baking-dish.

1 teaspoon Butter in 9 x 9 ceramic or glass baking dish. Microwave for 20 seconds and spread the butter on the bottom and sides of the dish.

Arrange in the bottom on the dish:

1/2 cup Fresh or Canned Pineapple Sliced & 1/2 cup dried Cranberries

Drain juice. Place Pineapple slices in the bottom of the pan. Sprinkle Cranberries between the slices.

1 Tablespoon Coconut Palm Sugar – Sprinkle evenly on the top of the fruits. Pour the blended batter on top and bake in preheated oven. Remove from oven and cool 5 minutes. Flip the cake onto a serving plate.

Bake 350 degrees or 175c for 40 minutes.

Serving size: 1/9th Calories = 141   Carbs = 22g   Protein = 4.6g   Fat = 0g

3.

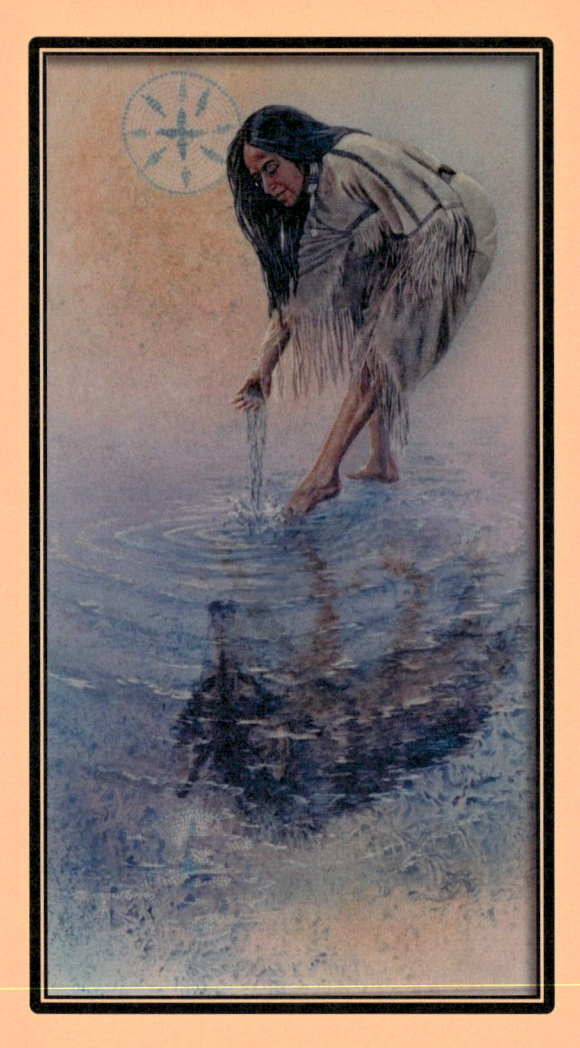

STILL WATERS 10 x 20 Giclee on Canvas
Signed and Numbered Limited Edition of 95

She sees a reflection of her spirit, the wolf.
She is the communicator, the traveler, the pathfinder
and the teacher.

4.

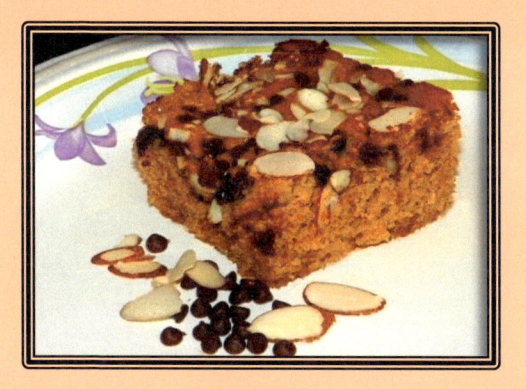

ALMOND CHOCOLATE CHIP CAKE

Pre-heat oven to 350 degrees

In a blender add the following and blend until smooth and creamy:

4 large Eggs

1 can - rinsed /drained Chick Peas (Garbanzo Beans) 15 oz. can

3/4 cup Coconut Palm Sugar

1 Tablespoon Almond Extract

2 teaspoons Baking Powder

1/4 cup Enjoy Life Mini Chocolate Chips (Add last- blend lightly)

    1 teaspoon Butter in 9 x 9 ceramic or glass baking dish. Microwave for 20 seconds and spread the butter on the bottom and sides of the dish. Pour blended batter into the dish. Sprinkle toppings over raw batter and place in pre-heated oven.

Toppings:

1/4 cup unsalted Slivered Almonds

2 Tablespoons Enjoy Life Mini Chocolate Chips

Bake 350 degrees or 175c for 40 minutes.

Cake 1/9th   Calories = 130 Carbs = 24g Protein = 4.6g Fat = 0g
Topping 1/9th Calories = 56 Carbs = 6g   Protein = 3g   Fat = 3.5g

5.

On Gossamer Wings – Stormy's Story

We met at an art show in Boulder, Co and as we were talking, Stormy was asking me about some of the meanings behind the Native themes of my work. I said, I'd explain but, why was the blonde, blue-eyed white woman telling her about Indians. She shared that she was raised from birth in a Catholic Orphanage. She had recently found her birth mother and knew she was Mountain Ute. I was raised on Reservations in AZ and SD. One of the Native families that I wanted Stormy to meet were the Bald Eagles. When they finally met at Artist Ride in South Dakota, David Bald Eagle and his wife Josie took Stormy into their hearts. David announced in 1995, that Stormy would be adopted as a family member and given a Lakota name the following year. Josie placed a star quilt around Stormy; welcomed her to their family and invited us to her naming ceremony. Stormy's given name is Mary and her nickname was Stormy. In a phone conversation with Stormy one time, she said "Kathy one of my biggest problems is that I don't know who I am". I said, "You are Stormy". She replied that that wasn't really her name. That was just a nickname. A few hours before the naming ceremony, Stormy was to meet with the Shaman. They would talk awhile, and then he would tell her, her Lakota name and what it means in English. The medicine man was told nothing about her including her nickname, Stormy. The Lakota name would be announced through the song by the singers during the ceremony. It sprinkled off and on through-out the day and finally the time came for the adoption and naming ceremony. We, who didn't speak Lakota, were told after the song, that Stormy's new name was O Si Ci Ca Win, (O See Chee Cha Wheen) which means Storm Woman.
The medicine man agreed after talking with her that this was her correct name. We danced in the mud in celebration and it continued to rain softly. Later as I hugged Stormy, I said, "Stormy, why couldn't you be named Sunny!"

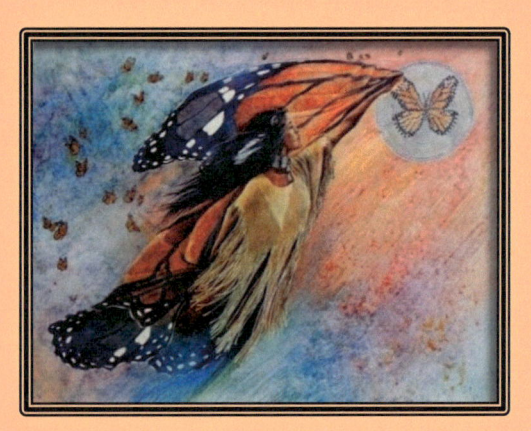

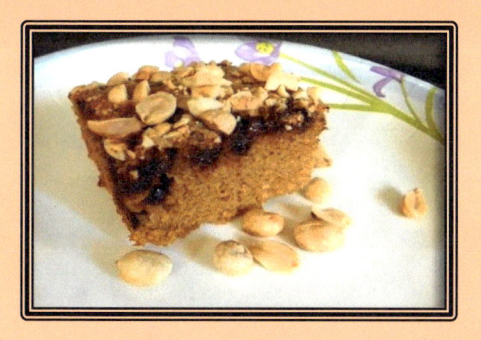

PEANUT BUTTER CHOCOLATE CHIP CAKE

Pre-heat oven to 350 degrees

In a blender add the following and blend until smooth and creamy:

4 large Eggs
1 can - rinsed /drained Chick Peas (Garbanzo Beans) 15 oz. can
3/4 cup Coconut Palm Sugar
1 Tablespoon Vanilla Extract
1/2 cup natural creamy or chunky Peanut Butter
2 teaspoons Baking Powder

1 teaspoon Butter in 9 x 9 ceramic or glass baking dish. Microwave for 20 seconds and spread the butter on the bottom and sides of the dish. Sprinkle toppings evenly on top of the raw batter. Pat down into the raw batter and place in the pre-heated oven.

Toppings
1/4 cup chopped unsalted Peanuts
1/4 cup Enjoy Life Mini Chocolate Chips

Bake 350 degrees or 175c for 40 minutes.

Cake 1/9th   Calories = 178   Carbs = 24g   Protein = 7g   Fat = 7g
Topping 1/9th Calories = 78   Carbs = 8g   Protein = 1g   Fat = 3.5g

7.

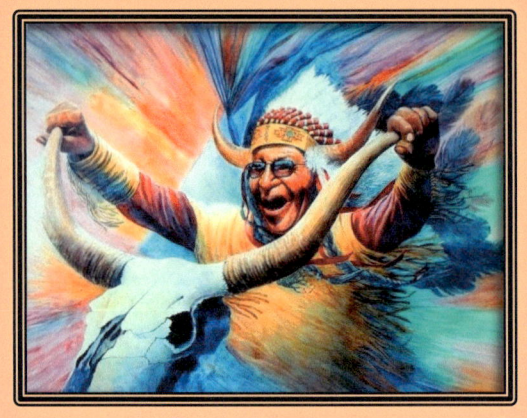

Do'in 80

My friend David Bald Eagle was 83 years young when I photographed him riding on a four-wheeler. We were at a gathering of Cowboys, Indians, Mountain men and artists in South Dakota and all week David's children and grandchildren had been riding back and forth from their Tee pee to various photo locations. On the last day, as we were all packing up to go home, I asked David when he was going to get to ride. I wanted to photograph him with his regalia and his full Buffalo Bonnet. He was happy to do it. The idea began to take on a life of its own. We added the Sunglasses and later put on the long horn skull for handle bars. In my painting I wanted to capture David's energy and to capture the spirit of the ride. We had a ball as he drove full speed all over the prairie, through the tee pees and with the little ones screaming and scattering as he went. I want to be Do' In 80 like this.

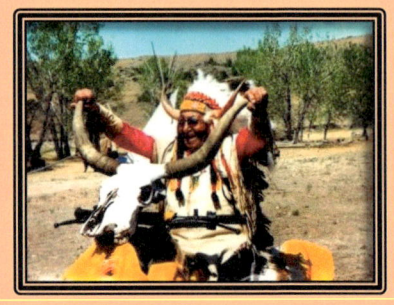

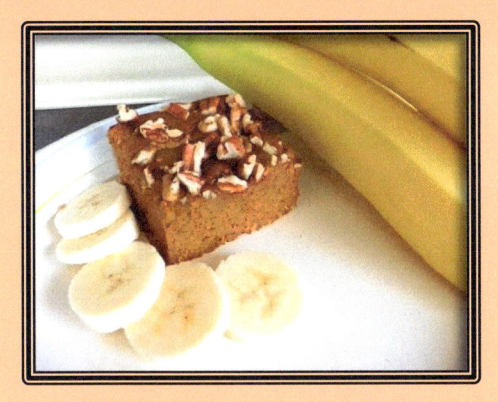

BANANA NUT BREAD
Pre-heat oven to 350 degrees
In a blender add the following and blend until smooth and creamy:

4 large Eggs

1 can - rinsed /drained Chick Peas (Garbanzo Beans) 15 oz. size

3/4 cup Coconut Palm Sugar

1 Tablespoon Vanilla Extract

1 1/2 Large ripe peeled Bananas

2 teaspoons Baking Powder

1 teaspoon Butter in 9 x 9 ceramic or glass baking dish. Microwave for 20 seconds and spread the butter on the bottom and sides of the dish. Sprinkle toppings evenly on top of the raw batter and place in the pre-heated oven.

Toppings:

1/2 cup chopped Pecans

1 Tablespoon Coconut Palm Sugar

Bake 350 degrees or 175c for 45 minutes.

Slice 1/9th   Calories = 138   Carbs = 25g   Protein = 4.6g   Fat = 0g
Topping 1/9th Calories = 47   Carbs = 2g   Protein = 4g   Fat = 3g

9.

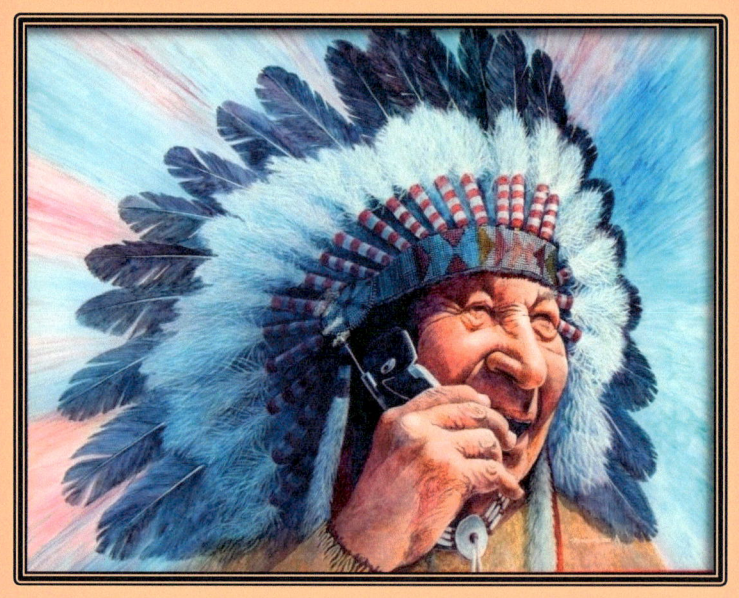

Wanan Namayanhun Huwo? Original 24 x 32

Chief David Bald Eagle has been a friend of mine since the 1980's. I have made many paintings of David and his family members. We met at Artist Ride in South Dakota where he was a model for the many artists that attend. We had finished a pretty long hot day of photography and David was dressed in his eagle feather bonnet and beaded shirt and pants that his wife Josee had made for him. He had a beautiful hand-quilted leather bag that was decorated with dyed porcupine quills. As we were walking from his tepee to my camp, his bag started buzzing. I said, David, "What is that noise?" He reached in the quilted bag and pulled out his cell phone. The idea hit like a hammer. David was willing to pose for me, but I like to keep it real. As he held the cell phone to his ear, I decided to make him laugh by bringing up something that had happened that Spring….. "David! It's Josee on the phone…the truck broke down in Deadwood and she needs a new Alternator." That tickled his funny bone and he cracked up laughing and I got what I was looking for. To embellish my tall tale a bit further, I added smoke signals coming out of the antenna. Four puffs for a GOOD SIGNAL! David helped me name this painting, by telling me the Lakota way to say "Can you hear me now?" Wanan Namayanhun Huwo? (Waana Naama Ya Hun Hoo Wo?)

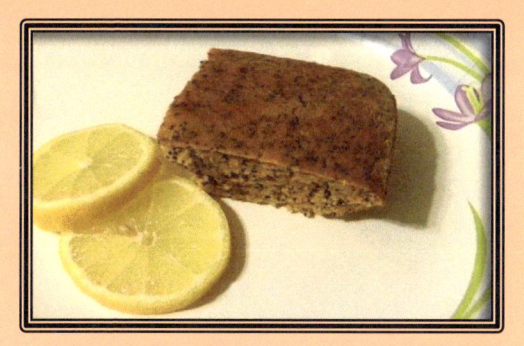

LEMON POPPY SEED CAKE
Pre-heat oven to 350 degrees

1/2 Lemon (wash thoroughly with soap & water, rinsed well) Trim off end, slice and remove any seeds. Place lemon with peel in the blender. Blend thoroughly and add eggs.

4 large Eggs - Blend thoroughly and add the rest of the ingredients.

1 can - rinsed /drained Chick Peas (Garbanzo Beans) 15 oz. size

3/4 cup Coconut Palm Sugar

1 Tablespoon Lemon Extract

2 teaspoons Baking powder

2 Tablespoons Poppy Seeds - Stir for a few seconds after the batter is well blended.

1 teaspoon Butter in a 9 x 9 ceramic or Pyrex baking dish. Microwave for 20 seconds and spread the butter on the bottom and sides of the dish. Sprinkle toppings evenly on top of the raw batter and place in the pre-heated oven.

Toppings:
1 Tablespoon Poppy Seeds
1 Tablespoon Coconut Palm Sugar
Bake 350 degrees or 175c for 45 minutes.

Cake 1/9th Calories = 119   Carbs = 20g   Protein = 4.6g   Fat = 0g
Topping 1/9th Calories = 7   Carbs = 1g   Protein = 0g   Fat = 0g

11.

The donkey's name is Rambo and he is full of mischief. I'm sure that if he had a chance to nibble on Geraniums, he would have taken the opportunity. The window and Geraniums were at the Lundeen Inn of The Arts Gallery in Las Cruces, NM. Rambo was in Colorado, but it sure made a good story!

The Mad Hatter-Giclee prints on Canvas 10 x 8 limited edition of 95 Signed and Numbered

Window of Opportunity
Original 48 x 24 Acrylic on Canvas

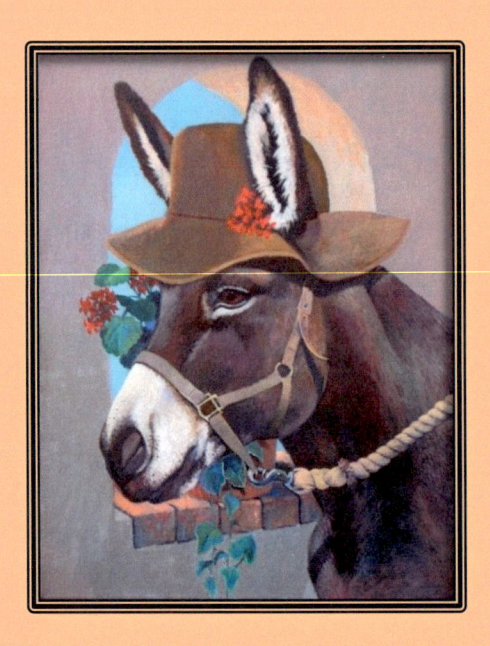

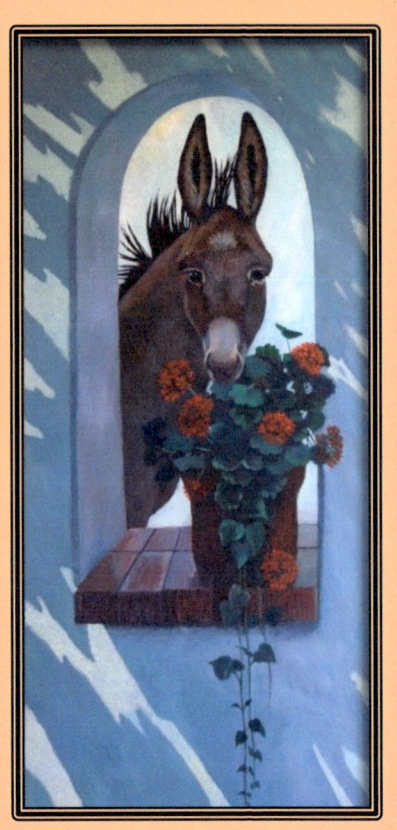

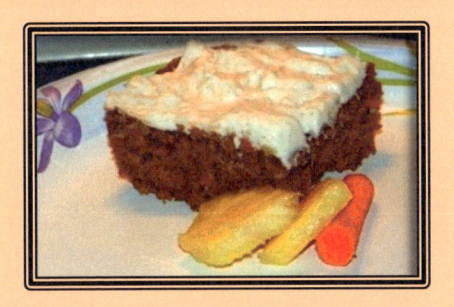

SPICY CARROT CAKE
Pre-heat oven to 350 degrees

1 cup Baby Carrots (chop carrots fine in the blender and save to a dish)
In the blender add the following and blend until smooth and creamy:
4 large Eggs
1 can - rinsed /drained Chick Peas (Garbanzo Beans) 15 oz. size
3/4 cup Coconut Palm Sugar
1 Tablespoon Vanilla Extract
2 teaspoons Baking Powder
2 teaspoons Cinnamon

After the batter is blended smooth, add the **Chopped Carrots** and blend on low for a few seconds to stir the carrots into the batter.

1 teaspoon Butter in a 9 x 9 ceramic or Pyrex baking dish. Microwave for 20 seconds and spread the butter. Pour batter into dish and place in the pre-heated oven.

Bake 350 degrees or 175c for 40 minutes.

Frosting: Whip with mixer on high for several minutes – spread on cooled cake.

4 oz. Cream Cheese (at room temperature)
1 Tablespoon Honey
1 teaspoon Vanilla
1/2 cup crushed Pineapple (thoroughly drained)

Slice 1/9th   Calories = 129   Carbs = 23g   Protein = 4.6g   Fat = 0g
Frosting 1/9th   Calories = 58   Carbs = 3.5g   Protein = 1g   Fat = 4.4g

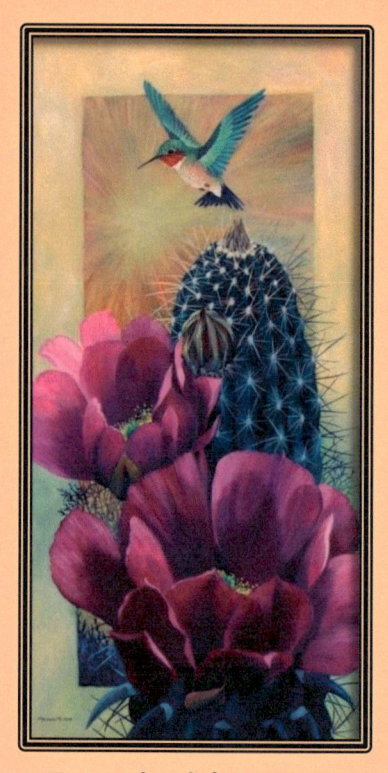

13.

Hedge Hog Cactus are part of the natural landscape around our house in New Mexico. The beautiful bright pink flowers attract many hummingbirds most common in our area are the Broad Tail Hummers. We maintain feeders and I can get good photos of these tiny aerial acrobats. Native Americans often refer to them as the littlest warriors as they seem to fear nothing.

The Lady or The Tiger- The hummer in The Lady or The Tiger is a female that is easily spotted by the tips of white on her tail and little or no red on her throat. Giclee on canvas limited edition of 95
Signed and Numbered 10 x 8

Pretty in Pink 24 x 12
A male Broad Tail Hummer at the top of Hedge Hog Cactus. Giclee on canvas limited edition of 95 Signed and Numbered

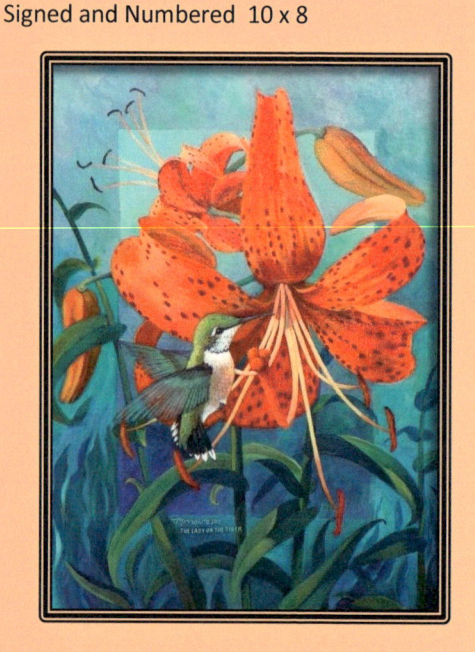

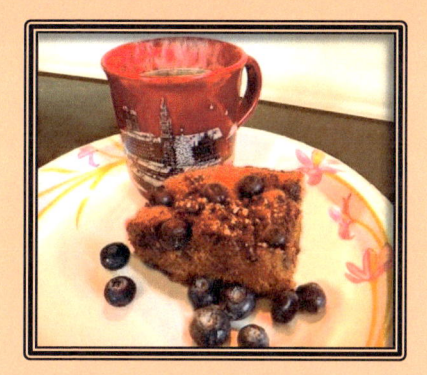

BLUEBERRY COFFEE CAKE

Pre-heat oven to 350 degrees

In a blender add the following and blend until smooth and creamy:

4 Large Eggs

1 can - rinsed /drained Chick Peas (Garbanzo Beans) 15 oz. size

3/4 cup Coconut Palm Sugar

1 Tablespoon Vanilla Extract

2 teaspoons Cinnamon

2 teaspoons Baking Powder

1 teaspoon Butter in a 9 x 9 ceramic or Pyrex baking dish. Microwave for 20 seconds and spread the butter on the bottom and sides of the dish. Sprinkle toppings evenly on top of the raw batter and place in the pre-heated oven

1/2 cup fresh or frozen Blueberries - sprinkle on top of the raw batter and stir berries down into batter with a fork.

Toppings:

1/2 Cup Chopped Pecans + 1/4 cup Blueberries

1 teaspoon Cinnamon + 1 Tablespoon Coconut Sugar - Pulse in the blender for 3 seconds spread evenly on top of raw batter. sprinkle **1/2 cup Blueberries** on top. Place in pre-heated oven.

Bake 350 degrees or 175c for 45 minutes.

Slice 1/9th   Calories = 125   Carbs = 22g   Protein = 4.6g   Fat = 0g

Toppings: Calories = 54   Carbs =3.5g   Protein =0g   Fat = 0g

15.

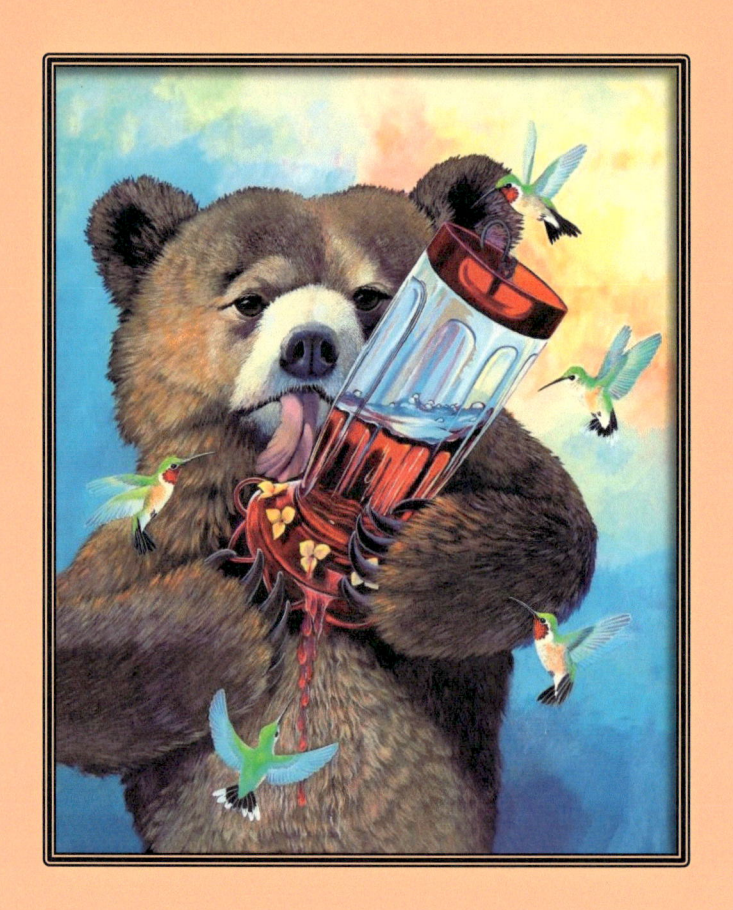

Sugar Bear 12 x 16

Last summer, I was doing a show at the Tanner Tradition Gallery in Ruidoso, NM. One morning a bear took out all their hummingbird feeders and the next day we saw a Mama Black bear and two cubs cross the road and walk right through the gallery parking lot headed for a little stream just behind the gallery. What a sight!
All of that inspired "Sugar Bear". A baby Black Bear is raiding the hummingbird feeder and boy are those little birds mad!

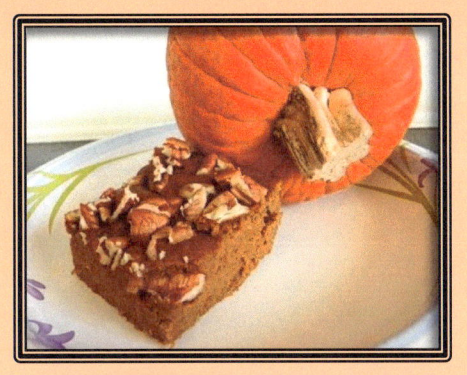

PUMPKIN NUT BREAD

Pre-heat oven to 350 degrees

In a blender add the following and blend until smooth and creamy:

4 large Eggs
1 can - rinsed /drained Chick Peas (Garbanzo Beans) 15 oz. size
3/4 cup Coconut Palm Sugar
1/2 can Pumpkin (1/2 15 oz. canned Pumpkin – freeze the rest)
1 Tablespoon Cinnamon
1/2 teaspoon Ground Ginger
1/4 teaspoon Nutmeg
1/4 teaspoon Allspice
2 teaspoons Baking Powder

1 teaspoon Butter in a 9 x 9 ceramic or Pyrex baking dish. Microwave for 20 seconds and spread the butter on the bottom and sides of the dish. Pour blended batter into buttered baking dish. Sprinkle topping on the raw batter.

Topping:
1 Tablespoon Coconut Palm Sugar + 1 teaspoon Cinnamon
1/2 cup chopped Pecans   Chop in blender a few seconds.
Bake 350 degrees or 175c for 45 minutes.

Slice 1/9th   Calories = 121   Carbs = 20g   Protein = 4.6g   Fat = 0g
Topping 19th Calories = 42   Carbs = 1g   Protein = 4g   Fat = 0g

17.

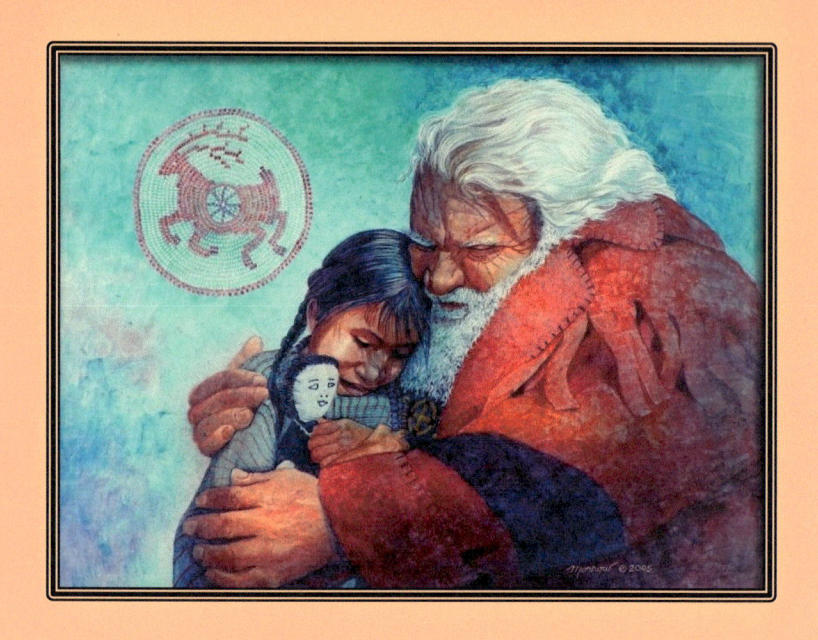

Navajo Barbie 16 x 20 Original Painting on Clay Board

Little Alyssia was the shy-est child I have ever seen. We spent a day trying to get her to relate to Santa, "Pilgrim" and it was- No go. I told her that my Navajo doll's name was Alyssia. Jay told her all about the elf at the North Pole, named Alyssia, who put the clothes on all the Barbie dolls. Alyssia was not impressed with our tall tales.   As luck would have it, my camera was on the fritz and the photos I took of her and Jay that day were all over exposed. Another artist helped me figure out the camera setting problem and we were good for the next day I did manage to get a few pictures, but my camera was acting up and I didn't want to cause her anymore discomfort by continuing on.
For the rest of the story read . . . . .
						Santa's Secret – (Page 19)

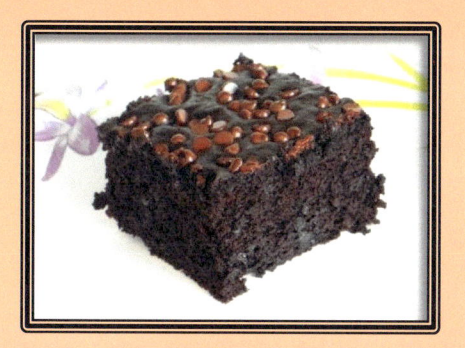

THE CHOCOLATE LADY'S CAKE

Pre-heat oven to 350 degrees
In a blender add the following and blend until smooth and creamy:

4 large Eggs
1 can - rinsed/drained Chick Peas (Garbanzo Beans) 15 oz. size
3/4 cup Coconut Palm Sugar
1 Tablespoon Vanilla Extract
1/4 cup Cocoa Powder (unsweetened Hershey's Dark)
4 oz. Natural Applesauce (unsweetened individual serving)
2 teaspoon Baking Powder
1/2 cup Enjoy Chocolate Mini Chips (Add last and stir lightly into well blended batter)

1 teaspoon Butter in a 9 x 9 ceramic or Pyrex baking dish. Microwave for 20 seconds and spread the butter on the bottom and sides of the dish.
Pour blended batter into buttered baking dish.
Sprinkle top of raw batter with Chocolate chips and almonds.

Toppings:
1/4 cup Enjoy Life Mini Chocolate Chips

Bake 350 degrees or 175c for 40 minutes.

Slice 1/9th   Calories = 189   Carbs = 30g   Protein = 5.6g   Fat = 4.5g
Topping 1/9th Calories =33   Carbs = 4g   Protein = .5g   Fat = 2g

19.

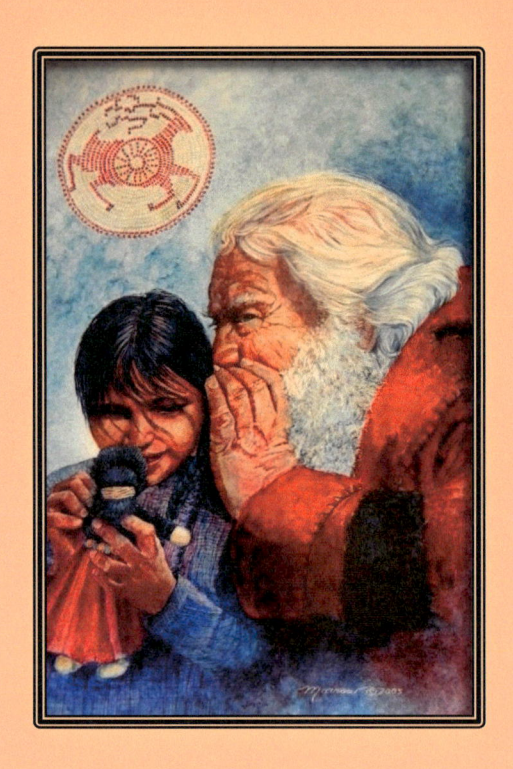

Santa's Secret 20 x 16 Original Painting on Clay Board

. . . . that night, I went to all the camps on the ranch that are scattered up and down the Cheyenne River. You see I am the "Chocolate Lady." Every year for about 10 years I have gone around in the evening with a giant bag of chocolate to pass out to all the good little girls and boys. And some not so little and some not so good!

When I got to Alyssia's family camp, I gave everyone a chocolate, her mom and brothers and sisters too but I told Alyssia she was my most favorite model and she got 4 chocolates! That girl was my best buddy the next day and we got some beautiful images from her. Jay was whispering to her that she got 4 chocolates and HE didn't get any!!!. You can see the coy little smile on her face. Thought you would like to know the story behind the Mona Lisa smile!

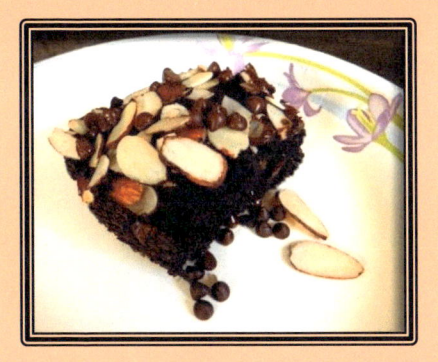

CHOCOLATE ALMOND CAKE

Pre-heat oven to 350 degrees

In a blender add the following and blend until smooth and creamy:

4 large Eggs
1 can - rinsed /drained Chick Peas (Garbanzo Beans) 15 oz. size
3/4 cup coconut Palm Sugar
1 Tablespoon Almond Extract
1/4 cup Cocoa Powder – (Unsweetened Hershey's Dark)
4 oz. Natural Applesauce (unsweetened individual serving)
2 teaspoons Baking Powder
1/2 cup Enjoy Life Mini Chocolate Chips (Add last and stir lightly into well blended batter)

1 teaspoon Butter in a 9 x 9 ceramic or Pyrex baking dish Microwave for 20 seconds and spread the butter on the bottom and sides of the dish.

Pour blended batter into buttered baking dish.

Toppings: Sprinkle on top of batter and place in pre-heated oven.
1/4 cup sliced unsalted almonds
1/4 cup Enjoy Life Mini Chocolate Chips

Bake 350 degrees or 175c for 40 minutes.

Slice 1/9th   Calories = 190   Carbs = 30g   Protein =5.6g   Fat = 0g
Topping 1/9th Calories = 55   Carbs = 5g   Protein = 2.5g   Fat = 3.5g

21.

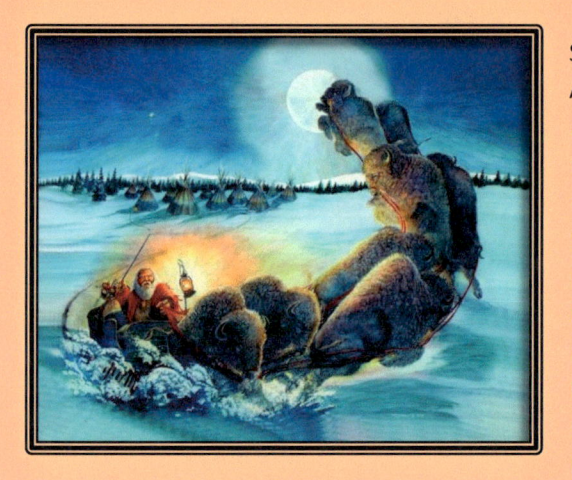

Santa is being pulled by American Bison (buffalo) as he cracks his buggy-whip with a magic spark on its tip. He has left the Lakota Village of Tee Pees and he is about to head out into the night. The Star of Bethlehem leads the way as he carries a sack in his antique sleigh. The

Tatanka Christmas 18 x 24

sack is filled with Lakota, Navajo and Apache Dolls, Bows and Arrows and a small stuffed Buffalo doll. I was going to photograph 2600 buffalo at the Triple 7 Ranch and my Santa friend, Jay Lewis at the Shearer Ranch in South Dakota. I have made a Santa painting every year for many years with Jay and ideas had always come easily. This time I was stuck. Dry as a bone. Not an idea in sight. Then I went to sleep and had the wildest dream. You can see it for yourself, as I was floating in the air and watching Santa driving his mighty steeds from the village, across the snow and into the moonlit night. I could feel the snow flying in my face. When I woke, I jotted it all down in a quick sketch. I saw Jay and told him all about the dream. We began assembling all the pieces. The sleigh was at the ranch. The cowboys helped me prop it up in front with logs so it would look like it was about to take off. Jay had a buggy whip and a bag and I gathered all my dolls and toys to fill the opening. I was telling the ranchers son, Garrett that I was up in the air. He asked how high up? Then came around with a front end loader and I got in the bucket and was lifted about 10 ft. to the perfect angle! We waited for twilight and lit the scene with a Coleman lantern. The next day we went to the Triple 7 and photographed buffalo. I got a set of bulls down in a valley. I got bulls at eye level and where was I going to get the flying ones? As we rounded a corner in the pickup, there were two bulls standing on a ledge above us. One tossed his head in the air and I swear they looked like they were flying. This painting is literally a dream come true.

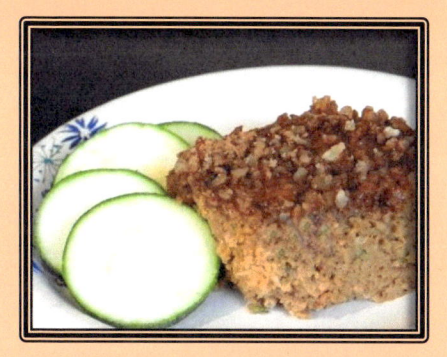

ZUCCINI NUT BREAD

Pre-heat oven to 350 degrees

1/2 Cup chopped fresh Zucchini Chop in blender for a few seconds and reserve in a bowl for later

In a blender add the following and blend until smooth and creamy:

4 large Eggs

1 can - rinsed /drained Chick Peas (Garbanzo Beans) 15 oz. size

3/4 cup Coconut Palm Sugar

1 Tablespoon Vanilla Extract

2 teaspoons Cinnamon

2 teaspoon Baking powder

Add **Chopped Zucchini** last and blend a few seconds to stir in.

1 teaspoon Butter in a 9 x 9 ceramic or Pyrex baking dish. Microwave for 20 seconds and spread the butter Pour blended batter into buttered baking dish. Sprinkle top of batter with sugar and Pecans

1/2 cup chopped Pecans

1 Tablespoon Coconut Palm Sugar

Bake 350 degrees or 175c for 45minutes.

Slice 1/9th   Calories = 118   Carbs = 20g   Protein = 4.6g   Fat = 0g
Topping 1/9th Calories = 47   Carbs = 2g   Protein = 4g   Fat = 3g

23.

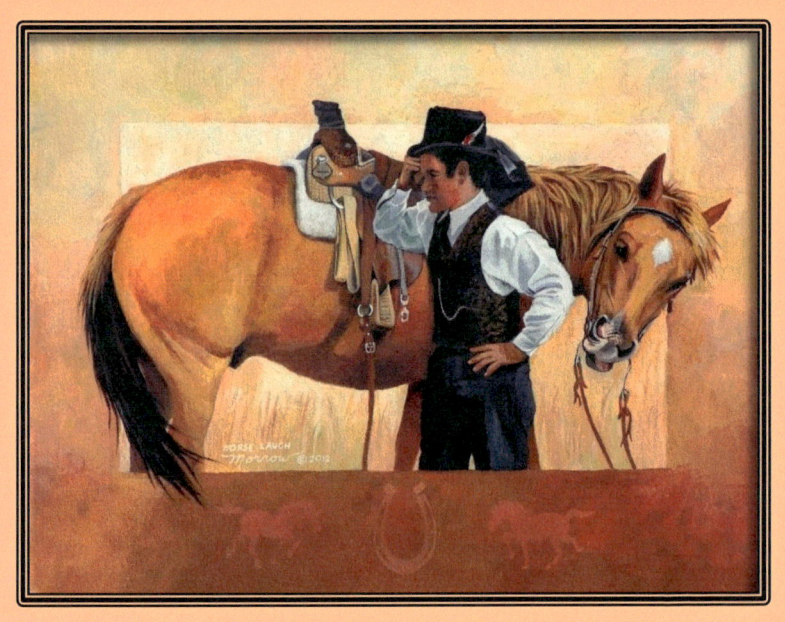

Horse Laugh 8 x 10 Limited Edition Giclee Prints on Canvas

Garrett Shearer is my model and boy did we have fun with this scene. He dressed as a "Dandy" or Dude and we started doing silly ideas with his horse, Stetson. I asked him to throw the saddle on backwards and he pretended to scratch his head as he looked puzzled. At that moment his horse was staring at the other horses across the pasture and I said it would be great if we could get the horse to turn and look at him like he was nuts. Garrett said, "I can do that!" Then he put some grass in his back pocket and Stetson turned his head and stretched out his lips to get the grass that was a little out of his reach. It looked just like Stetson was laughing!

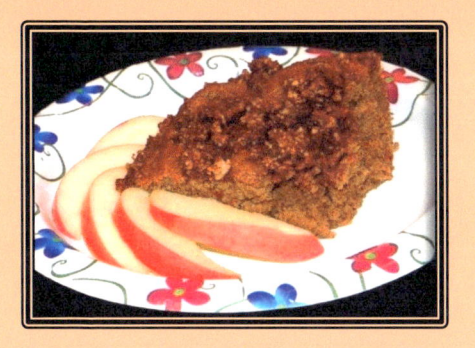

APPLE CRUMBLE CAKE

Pre-heat oven to 350 degrees

In a blender add the following and blend until smooth and creamy:

4 large Eggs
1 can - rinsed /drained Chick Peas (Garbanzo Beans) 15 oz. size
3/4 cup Coconut Palm Sugar
1 Tablespoon Vanilla Extract
1/2 Apple cut into pieces (Fuji, Gala or Granny)
1 Tablespoon Cinnamon
2 teaspoons Baking Powder

1 teaspoon Butter in a 9 x 9 ceramic or Pyrex baking dish. Microwave for 20 seconds and spread the butter. Pour blended batter into buttered baking dish. Sprinkle batter with sugar, pecans and apple topping.

Topping: (Chop in the blender a few seconds till crumbly)
1/2 cup chopped Pecans
1/4 cup Coconut Palm Sugar
1/2 Apple cut into pieces (Fuji, Gala or Granny)
1 teaspoon Cinnamon

Bake 350 degrees or 175c for 40 minutes.

Slice 1/9th   Calories = 122   Carbs = 21g   Protein = 4.6g   Fat = 0g
Topping 1/9th   Calories = 61   Carbs = 5g   Protein = 4g   Fat = 3g

25.

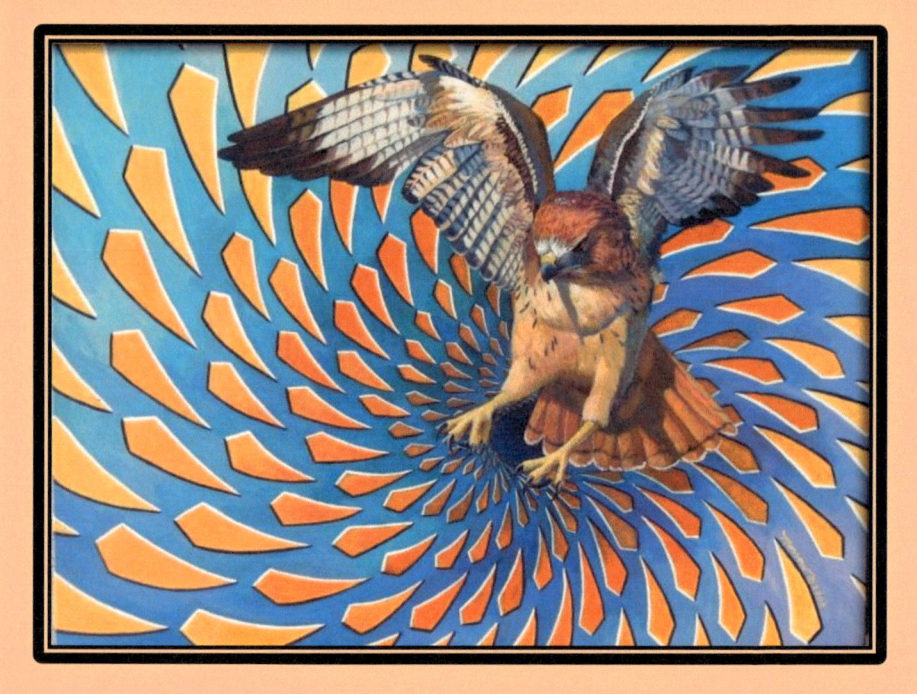

Sky Hawk – Optical Illusion,
18 x 24 Original Acrylic on Canvas with
Gallery Wrapped Edges

The Red Tail Hawk is flying through a moving vortex. I love playing with optical illusions and Sky Hawk is painted with a careful balance of medium, dark and light tones. The background design is painted in a way that creates an illusion of movement. By focusing only on the hawk you will begin to see the background rotate slowly counter clockwise. 5 % of the population are not able to see this illusion and there is no known reason why some don't see it. Once you do see the movement, you will always see it when you look at the painting.

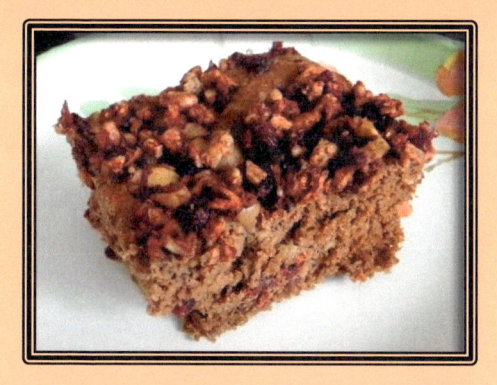

CRANBERRY NUT CAKE

Pre-heat oven to 350 degrees

In a blender add the following and blend until smooth and creamy:

- 4 large Eggs
- 1 can - rinsed /drained Chick Peas (Garbanzo Beans) 15 oz. size
- 1 Tablespoon Vanilla
- 1 Tablespoon Cinnamon
- 3/4 cup Coconut Palm Sugar
- 2 teaspoons Baking Powder
- 1/2 cup dried Cranberries (add last after batter is well blended and blend for a few seconds)

1 teaspoon Butter in a 9 x 9 ceramic or Pyrex baking dish. Microwave for 20 seconds and spread the butter. Pour blended batter into buttered baking dish. Sprinkle top of batter with Cinnamon, sugar, dried Cranberries and Apples.

Toppings: Chop in the blender for a few seconds:

- 1 teaspoon Cinnamon
- 1 Tablespoon Coconut Palm Sugar
- 1/4 cup dried Cranberries and 1/4 cup chopped pecans
- 1/2 Apple (cut into pieces)

Bake 350 degrees or 175c for 40 minutes.

Slice 1/9th   Calories = 138   Carbs = 25g   Protein = 4.6g   Fat = 0g

Topping 1/9th   Calories = 19   Carbs = 4g   Protein = 0g   Fat = 0g

27.

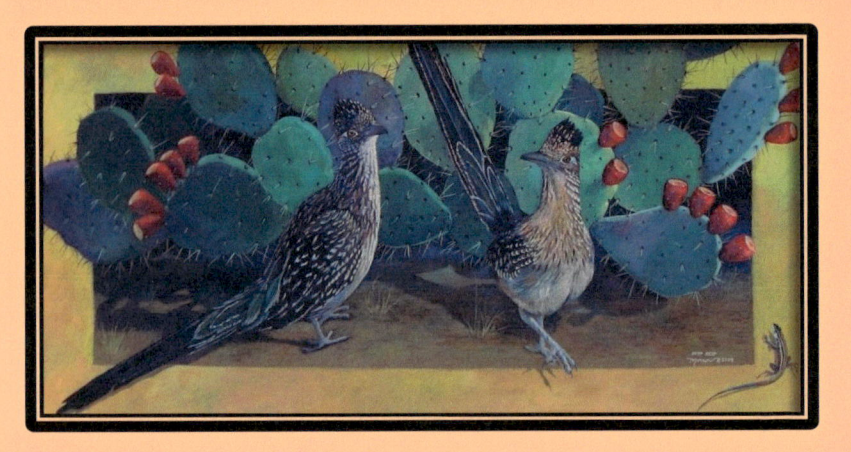

BEEP BEEP 12 x 24   Limited Edition Giclee Prints on canvas
These two roadrunners spent the spring and summer drinking from our dogs' water dish and dashing in and out of the yard, driving them nuts! It was easy to get good photos as they came up to my backdoor and were curious about what was inside.
I think the lizard might get away. What do you think?

Detail of Beep Beep

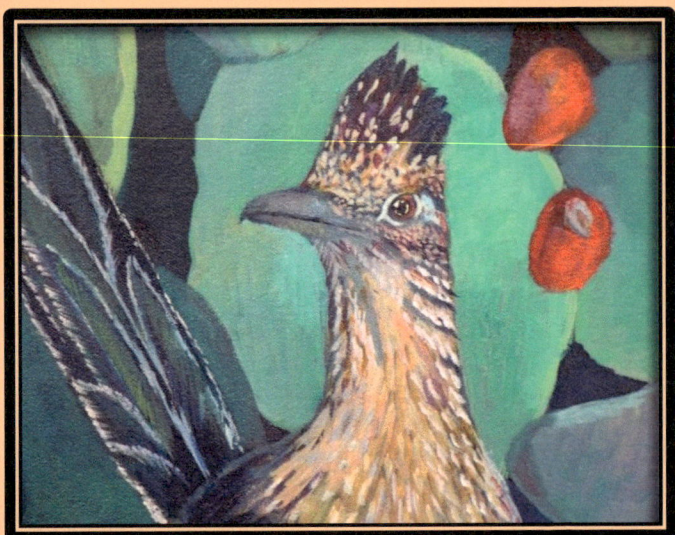

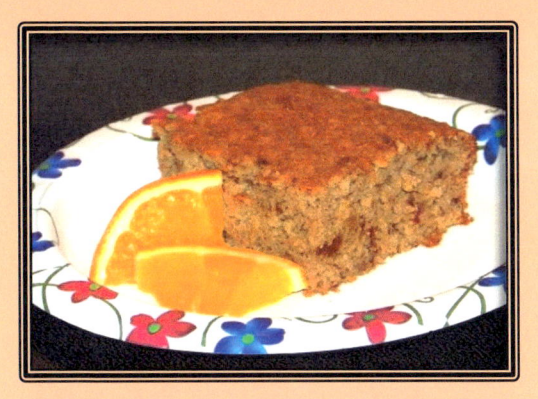

ORANGE DATE NUT BREAD
Pre-heat oven to 350 degrees

1/2 Medium Orange - wash thoroughly with soap & water, rinse well and trim off the end, slice and remove any seeds. Place orange with peel in the blender. Blend thoroughly and add eggs and continue blending.

Add remaining ingredients and blend until smooth and creamy:

4 large Eggs blend with orange and add the rest of the ingredients

1 can - rinsed /drained Chick Peas (Garbanzo Beans) 15 oz. size

1 Tablespoon Orange Extract

1/2 cup Coconut Palm Sugar

2 teaspoons Baking Powder

1/2 cup Pecans (Add nuts and dates last and blend for only a few seconds after the batter is well blended)

4 Large Medjool dates pitted and cut into pieces.

1 teaspoon Butter in a 9 x 9 ceramic or Pyrex baking dish. Microwave for 20 seconds and spread the butter. Pour blended batter into buttered baking dish.

Bake 350 degrees or 175c for 45 minutes.

Slice $1/9^{th}$ Calories = 150   Carbs = 17g   Protein = 8.6g   Fat = 3g

29.

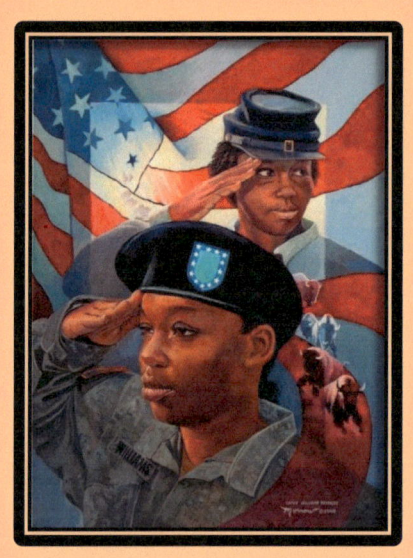

Cathy Williams Revealed 12 x 16

Signed and numbered limited edition on canvas of 95. Cathy Williams enlisted as a Buffalo Soldier in 1866 after she was freed as a slave. She enlisted under the name William Cathay and kept her identity as a female secret. She served for two years before leaving company A and began a new life as a successful business woman in Trinidad, Colorado.

Cathy Williams Revealed shows a female soldier proudly saluting. In the background, she is a Buffalo Soldier of 1866. The past and today are separated by a herd of running buffalo coming from the stars of the flag. Her history plays an important part of her own self-discovery and confidence as today's soldier. My model and friend, Monique, dressed up in army uniforms from the 1860's and 2010. We posed at sunset and then draped the American flag in front of the sunset to back light through the flag for a special effect. The buffalo running out to the sunburst toward the modern Cathy Williams are from the Triple 7 Ranch in South Dakota. I was behind a large cement barrier as the buffalo were running toward me into the next chute. Believe me when I say that was exciting filming!

30.

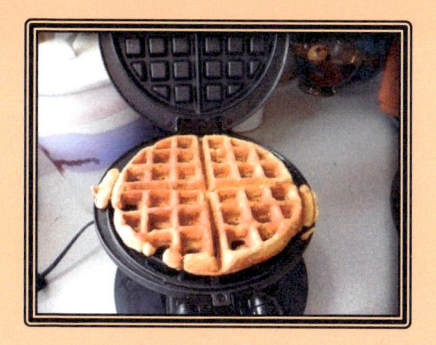

WAFFLES

In a blender add the following and blend until smooth and creamy:
4 large Eggs
1 can - rinsed /drained Chick Peas (Garbanzo Beans) 15 oz. size
1/4 cup Coconut Palm Sugar
1 Tablespoon Vanilla Extract
2 teaspoons Baking Powder

Pour 1/2 cup of batter onto a preheated waffle maker that has been lightly buttered. Close the lid, turn the handle and cook 2 minutes or until the steam stops coming out of the sides. Serve with favorite toppings or fresh fruit. Make 5-6 pancakes or waffles.

PANCAKES

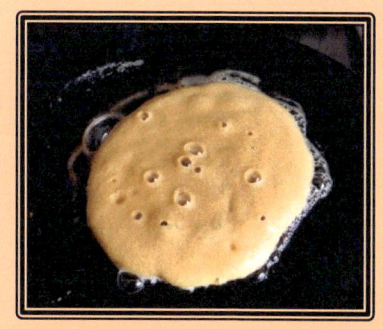

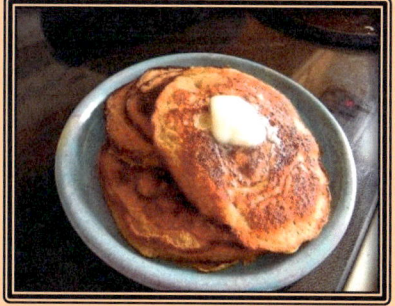

The Same recipe as above. Pour batter onto hot lightly buttered griddle. Turn after the bubbles on the surface start popping.

Makes 6   Calories = 142   Carbs = 15g   Protein =7.5g   Fat = 0g

31.

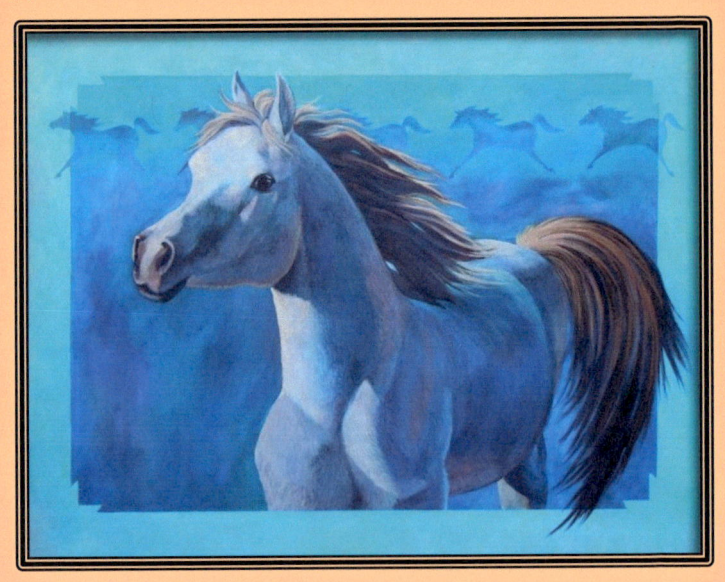

Ghost Dancing 36 x 48 Original Acrylic on Canvas. My friend, Don Parish, has modeled for me in many of my Buffalo Soldier paintings. He owns this lovely Arab named Ghost. I was out in the corral with Ghost right a sun rise and he was really showing off for the camera. He does look like he is dancing as he moves.

Don Parish and Ghost Dancing

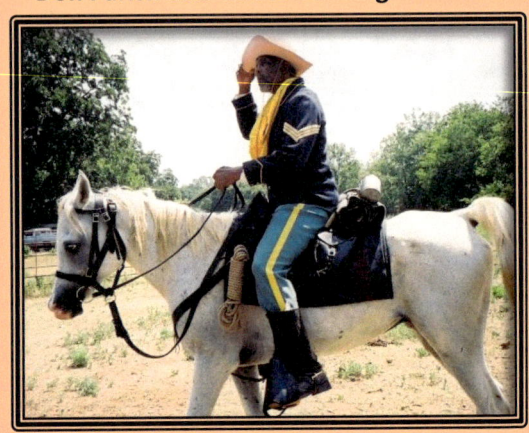

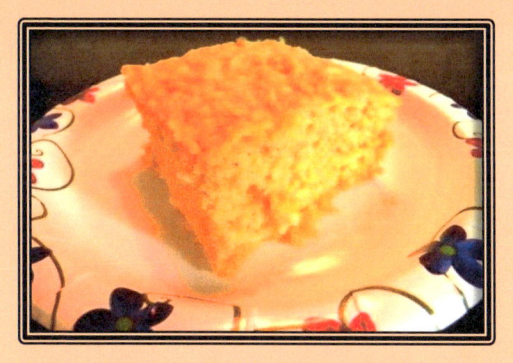

CHEESY CORNBREAD

Pre-heat oven to 350 degrees

In a blender add the following and blend until smooth and creamy:

- 4 large Eggs
- 1 can - rinsed /drained Chick Peas (Garbanzo Beans) 15 oz. size
- 1/4 cup Corn Meal
- 1 Tablespoon dried Onion Flakes
- 1 teaspoon Garlic Powder
- 1/2 cup frozen Corn
- 1/4 teaspoon Sea Salt
- 2 teaspoons Baking Powder
- 1/2 cup Cheddar Cheese

(Optional)

1 chopped Jalapeno or Green Chile Pepper. (Add Last-blend)

1 teaspoon Butter in a 9 x 9 ceramic or Pyrex baking dish. Microwave for 20 seconds and spread the butter. Pour blended batter into buttered baking dish. Sprinkle top of batter with 1/4 cup shredded Cheddar Cheese.

Bake 350 degrees or 175c for 45minutes.

Slice 1/9th Calories = 134   Carbs = 16g   Protein = 9g   Fat = 3g

(Sandwich Size slice)

Slice 1/6th Calories = 183   Carbs = 23g   Protein = 12g   Fat = 3g

33.

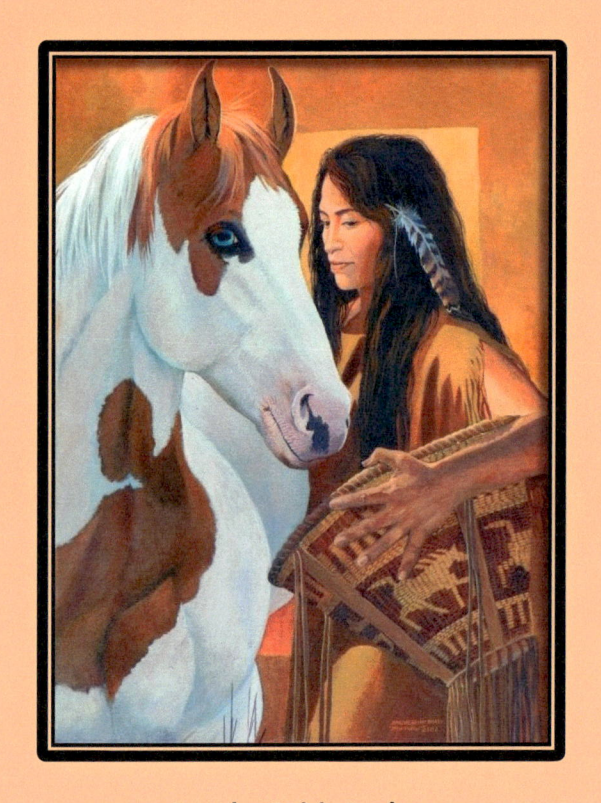

Apache Spirit Basket
Original Acrylic on canvas 24 x 18

Apache Burden Baskets are hand crafted from Cotton Wood bark and Mulberry sticks and are used as utility baskets to gather fruit, berries, herbs or nuts and to carry items. These baskets are still used in traditional Apache ceremonies today. The dark weave is the outside bark and the light weave is the inside of the bark. Apache women sometimes carried the basket against their backs with a strap across the forehead for support. The basket is wrapped with leather and decorated with numerous leather strips and tin cones that jingle when the basket is moved. This sound was said to ward off snakes as Apache women walked through the desert. My sister, Veronica who is Navajo and Apache was my model for Apache Spirit Basket. She is wearing a deerskin dress of my design and creation.

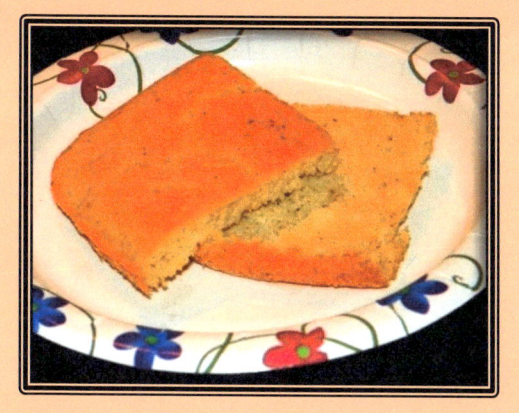

SANDWICH / HAMBURGER BUNS

Pre-heat oven to 350 degrees

In a blender add the following and blend until smooth and creamy:

- 4 large Eggs
- 1 can - rinsed /drained Chick Peas (Garbanzo Beans) 15 oz. size
- 1/4 cup Chobani Greek Yogurt (Plain)
- 1 Tablespoon dried Onion Flakes
- 1/2 teaspoon Garlic Powder
- 1/4 teaspoon Sea Salt
- 1/4 teaspoon Black Pepper
- 2 teaspoons Baking Powder

1 teaspoon Butter in a 9 x 9 ceramic or Pyrex baking dish. Microwave for 20 seconds and spread the butter. Pour blended batter into buttered baking dish.

Bake 350 degrees or 175c for 45 minutes.

Slice 1/9th Calories = 122   Carbs = 16g   Protein = 8g   Fat = 2g

(Sandwich Size slice)

Slice 1/6th Calories = 183   Carbs = 24g   Protein = 12g   Fat = 3g

35.

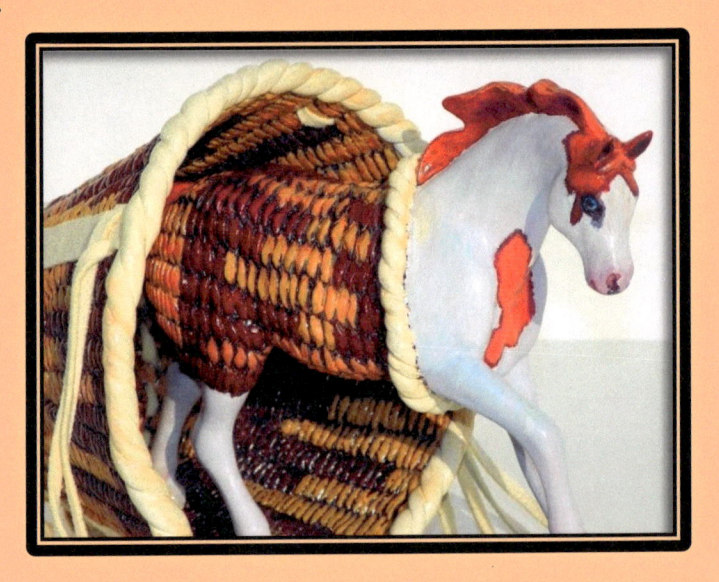

Apache Spirit Pony
6" x 9" Original Pony Design with sculpted Apache Burden Basket is a companion to Apache Spirit Basket on page 33.

Trail of Pained Ponies offered a miniature form that I enhance with additional sculpted designs. In this case replicating in great detail an Apache Burden Basket completed with real leather fringes and brass jingles. While I was working on this original, I had another name for it; "Basket Case" and I was almost a basket case before I finished this detailed sculpture. Below are images of the art work in progress.

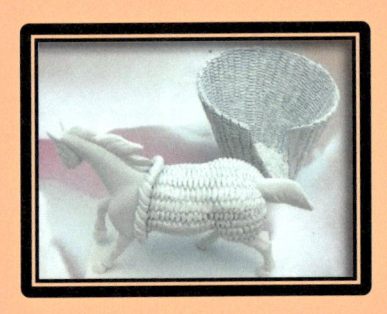

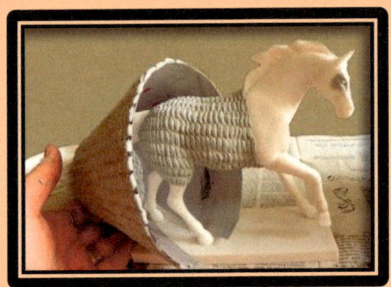

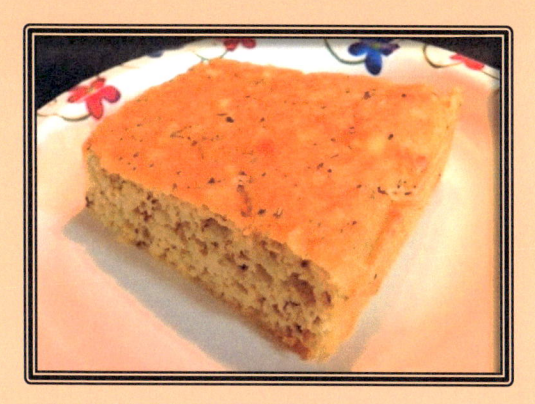

ITALIAN PARMESAN BREAD

Pre-heat oven to 350 degrees

In a blender add the following and blend until smooth and creamy:

2 oz. Fresh Parmesan Cheese Blend fine before adding the following:
4 large Eggs
1 can - rinsed /drained Chick Peas (Garbanzo Beans) 15 oz. size
1/4 cup Chobani Greek Yogurt (Plain)
1 Tablespoon dried Onion Flakes
1/2 teaspoon Garlic Powder
1 teaspoon Italian Herb mix (Basil, Oregano, Thyme)
1/4 teaspoon Sea Salt
2 teaspoons Baking Powder

1 teaspoon Butter in a 9 x 9 ceramic or Pyrex baking dish. Microwave for 20 seconds and spread the butter. Pour blended batter into buttered baking dish. Sprinkle top of raw batter with shredded Parmesan Cheese.
Bake 350 degrees or 175c for 45 minutes.

Slice 1/9th   Calories = 81   Carbs = 7g   Protein = 4.6g   Fat = 0g
(Sandwich Size slice)
Slice 1/6th   Calories = 123   Carbs = 11g   Protein = 7g   Fat = 0g

37.

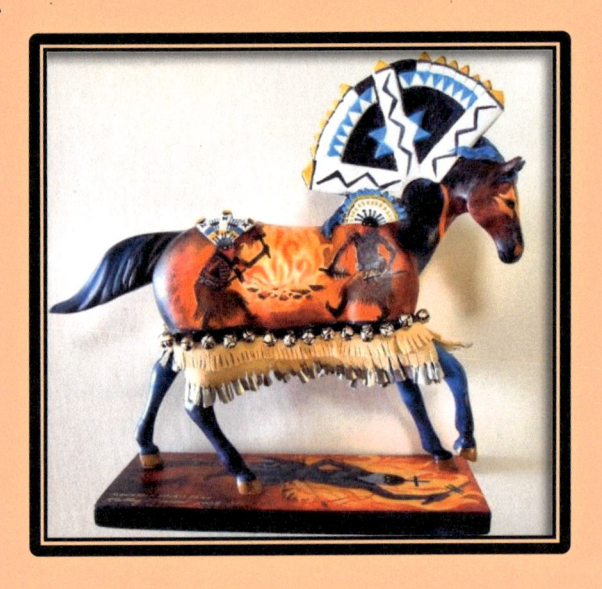

Apache Spirit Pony
6" x 9" Original Pony Design

My father organized and trained police forces on many Indian Reservations. When we lived on the San Carlos Apache Reservation, we attended coming of age ceremonials for young women and the Mountain Spirit Dancers were my inspiration for Apache Spirit Pony.

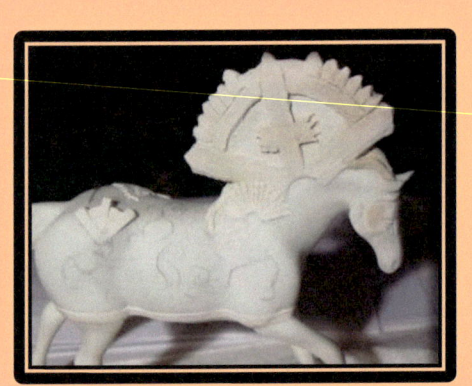

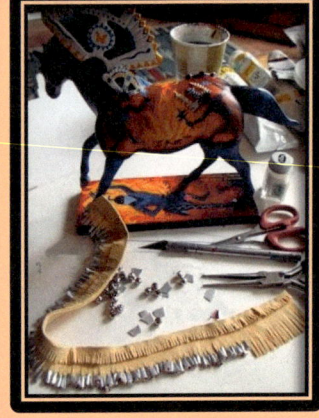

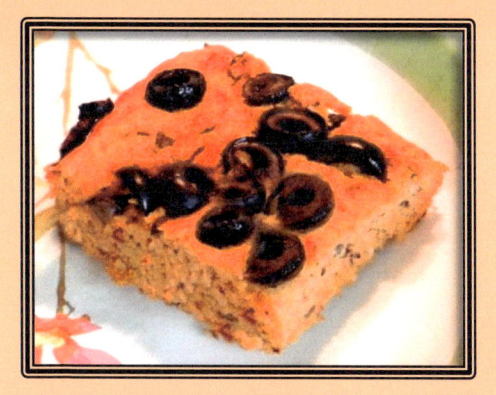

SUN DRIED TOMATO BREAD

Pre-heat oven to 350 degrees

In a blender add the following and blend until smooth and creamy:

2 oz. Fresh Parmesan Cheese Blend fine before adding the following:

4 large Eggs

1 can - rinsed /drained Chick Peas (Garbanzo Beans) 15 oz. size

1/4 cup Chobani Greek Yogurt (Plain)

1 Tablespoon dried Onion Flakes

1/2 teaspoon Garlic Powder

1/2 cup Sun Dried Tomatoes

1/4 teaspoon Sea Salt

2 teaspoons Baking Powder

25 Black Olives (about 1/2 15 oz. can) Blend last for just a few seconds

1 teaspoon Butter in a 9 x 9 ceramic or Pyrex baking dish. Microwave for 20 seconds and spread the butter. Pour blended batter into buttered baking dish. Sprinkle top of batter with Olives slices.

Topping: 25 Black Olives sliced

Bake 350 degrees or 175c for 45 minutes.

Slice $1/9^{th}$ Calories = 125   Carbs = 8g   Protein = 6g   Fat = 5g
(Sandwich Size slice)
Slice $1/6^{th}$ Calories = 190   Carbs = 12g   Protein = 9g   Fat = 8g

39.

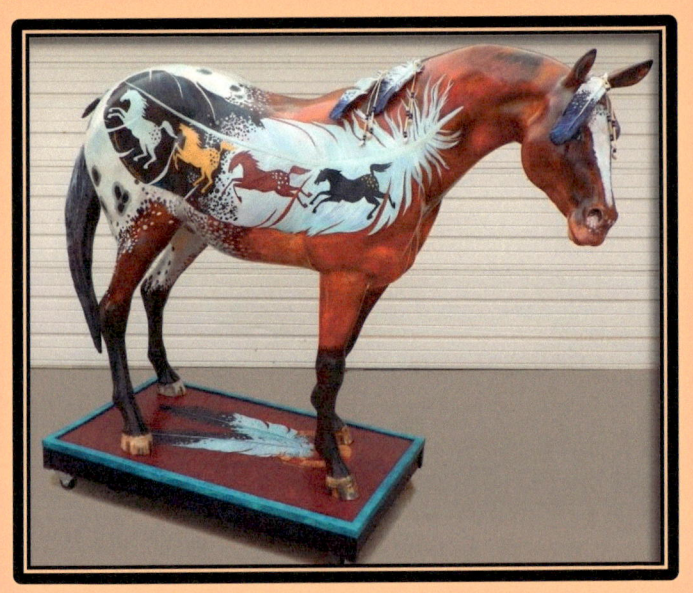

Horse Feathers
A life size pony custom painted for
Trail of Painted Ponies, a New Mexico Public Arts Project
was a powerful merge of businesses charities and artists for the benefit of the New Mexico community. In the first year of the projects conception, 120 life size horse sculptures were cast in a polyurethane resin. All artists began with the same sculpture as a blank canvas on which to create their art. Artists were allowed to alter the horses and many did. I sculpted and attached 7 eagle feathers to the mane and tail of Horse Feathers. Each artist was sponsored by a business and profit from the auction of the horses benefited New Mexico charities.

Horse Feathers combines the design patterns of the Appaloosa's Blanket on her back quarters with the spotted patterns in the eagle's feather. The four horses painted on the feather represent the rainbow of mankind: Red, Yellow, Black and White.

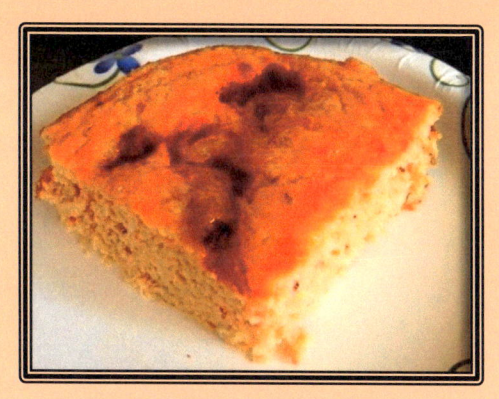

MEXICAN SALSA BREAD

Pre-heat oven to 350 degrees

In a blender add the following and blend until smooth and creamy:

  4 large Eggs
  1 can - rinsed /drained Chick Peas (Garbanzo Beans) 15 oz. size
  1/4 cup Chobani Greek Yogurt (Plain)
  1/2 cup shredded Cheddar Cheese (reserve about half for topping)
  1 Tablespoon dried Onion Flakes
  1/2 teaspoon Garlic Powder
  1/4 teaspoon Sea Salt
  2 teaspoons Baking Powder

1/2 cup 505 Red Salsa (add last and blend a few seconds)

1 teaspoon Butter in a 9 x 9 ceramic or Pyrex baking dish. Microwave for 20 seconds and spread the butter. Pour blended batter into buttered baking dish.

Topping: Sprinkle remainder Cheddar Cheese on top of raw batter and spoon a little salsa on for color.

Bake 350 degrees or 175c for 45 minutes.

Slice 1/9th Calories = 116   Carbs = 10g   Protein = 8g   Fat = 6.5g
(Sandwich Size slice)
Slice 1/6th Calories = 133   Carbs = 12g   Protein = 9g   Fat = 9g

41.

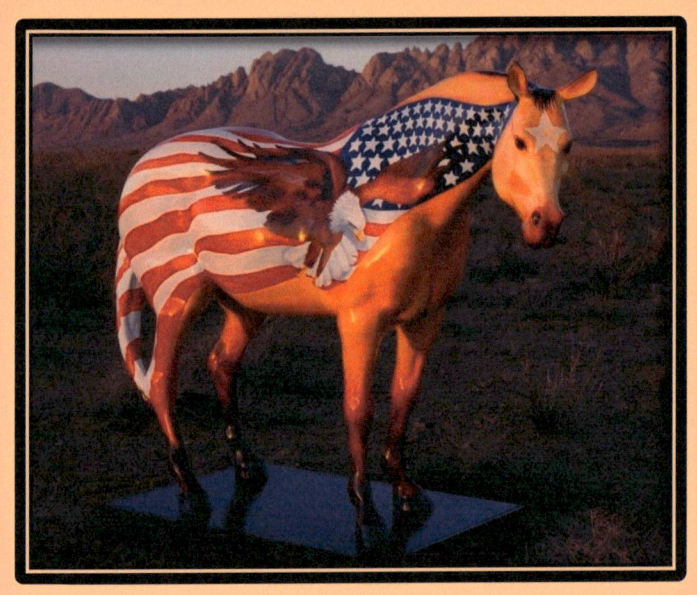

Give Me Wings
A life size pony custom painted for
Trail of Painted Ponies, a New Mexico Public Arts Project

The life size Give Me Wings is at 1st New Mexico Bank of Las Cruces in Las Cruces NM. Old Town Emporium sponsored Horse Feathers to benefit The Women's Community Association, an organization that offers safe haven for women and children who have experienced domestic violence. High Desert State Bank sponsored Give Me Wings to benefit Jardin de Los Ninos in Las Cruces, NM. Jardin educates and cares for young children of homeless and near homeless families while helping to them to recover.

Give Me Wings was inspired and designed after Sept 11th 2001. I wrote a poem on the pony that lines the edges of the flag.

I will not forget those who
Sacrificed on the altar of
Freedom, precious freedom,
Give Me Wings to soar beyond my dreams
And touch the Stars.   km

Give Me Wings was photographed with the beautiful Organ Mountains of Las Cruces, NM in the background. This is the view from my kitchen window.

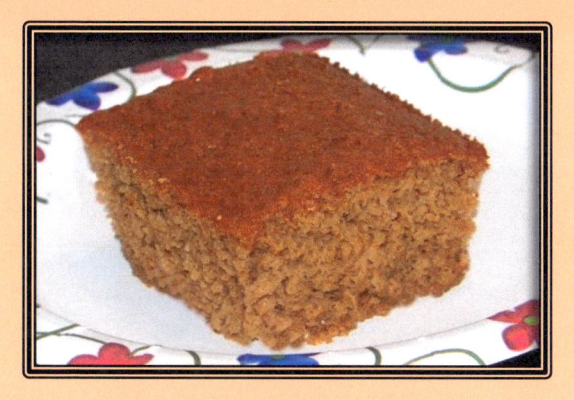

PLAIN VANILLA CAKE
Pre-heat oven to 350 degrees
In a blender add the following and blend until smooth and creamy:
- 4 large eggs
- 1 can - rinsed /drained Chick Peas (Garbanzo Beans) 15 oz. size
- 1 Tablespoon Vanilla
- 3/4 cup Coconut Palm Sugar
- 2 teaspoons Baking Powder

1 teaspoon Butter in a 9 x 9 ceramic or Pyrex baking dish. Microwave for 20 seconds and spread the butter. Pour blended batter into buttered baking dish.

(This cake is great with fresh fruit and whipped cream topping for a great shortcake)

Bake 350 degrees or 175c for 40 minutes.

Slice 1/9th   Calories = 115   Carbs = 16g   Protein = 8g   Fat = 2g

43.

THESE ARE A FEW OF MY FAVORITE THINGS:

Enjoy Life Mini Chocolate Chips: Produced in a Gluten Free Facility without Soy. They taste chocolaty and have a nice texture. Also available in chunks. It's almost impossible to find a good Chocolate that is soy free. Soy Lecithin is an emulsifier used in most chocolate Products in both US and Europe.

Organic Coconut Palm Sugar: Coconut Palm sugar is low on the glycemic index, high in nutrients. I found it to be a great substitute for cane sugar and it's not artificial. Carbohydrates are the same as cane sugar but blood sugar rises slowly instead of spiking.

Chobani Greek Yogurt: High protein and tastes like sour cream without the fat. Good substitute for Mayo in potato salad and other creamy dishes that call for sour cream.

505 Salsa: Red or Green The ingredients are just food, no preservatives or added chemicals or Natural Flavor.

Chick Peas or Garbanzo Beans: You can buy dried peas in 1 lb. bags and soak them in water for about 8 hours then cook them for 1 hour. Cool and bag them. ¾ cup to a freezer bag = One 15 oz. can without the liquid. Makes 4 portions.

The Ninja Blender: My new best friend in the kitchen! It's easy to use, easy to clean and powerful. It has two containers so I can chop the toppings in the small one and blend the batter in the large one.

AUTHOR'S NOTES:

It used to be rare to be gluten intolerant. About 1 person in 100,000 and it was difficult to diagnose. At the writing of this book, 2013, the level of Gluten intolerance is 1 in 106 people. Because it has become so common, grocery stores are expanding their product lines for Gluten free food. The breads, cakes and muffins are sometimes tasty but always more expensive than their counter parts in the regular bread aisle. I wanted to make recipes that were easy to assemble. Everything into a blender is my idea of easy. I wanted the recipes to be healthy and low glycemic for Diabetics. An added bonus is that most of the recipes are low in fat. If there is fat the main source are the added nuts and they can be optional.

Many Gluten free recipes for breads and cakes needed Xanthium Gum to keep the cake/bread from falling apart. Generally this is the "glue" that holds many food products together when Gluten's not there. I wanted to avoid these chemical additives and found that the basic bean and egg combination did not fall apart after baking.

In the blending stages, the recipe looks like it couldn't possibly work! When my grand-daughter, Nikki (who's been Type I Diabetic since she was 2 years old) and I baked our first cake, we were both skeptical about the batter and delighted when our cake came out of the oven smelling great and tasting wonderful. At that moment, I knew that this basic vanilla cake had potential to be so much more with a little imagination.

My art comes from my life experiences and most of my paintings have stories. I wanted to share just a few of these with you, as they are also . . . . . .

What's Cooking at Kathy Morrow's Studio.

What's Cooking at
Kathy Morrow's Studio
Published by
Kathy Morrow Studio
PO Box 1749
Mesilla Park, NM 88047
(800) 234-5641

www.kathymorrowstudio.com
art@kathymorrowstudio.com

Copyright 2013, Kathy Morrow Studio
All Rights Reserved